DASH DIET

Dash Diet: Easy and Healthy Recipes With Specific Nutritional Values & Meal Plans to Lose Weight & Improve Health

@ Peggy Hale

Published By Adam Gilbin

@ Peggy Hale

Dash Diet: Easy and Healthy Recipes With Specific Nutritional Values & Meal Plans to Lose Weight & Improve Health

All Right RESERVED

ISBN 978-1-990053-31-3

TABLE OF CONTENTS

Tuscan-Style Tuna Salad 1

Strawberry, Melon & Avocado Salad 2

Roast Chicken Dal 4

Spaghetti Squash With Chunky Tomato Sauce 6

Meatier Meatloaf 9

Pork Tenderloin Curry In Apple Cider 14

Clams Fettuccine 17

Strip Steak With Mushroom Whiskey Sauce.............. 19

Creamy Polenta With Veggies.................................... 21

Chicken Salad With Balsamic Vinaigrette And
Pineapple.. 24

Mushroom Oatmeal... 27

Eggs Mix 29

Carrot Oatmeal... 30

Dates And Millet Pudding 32

Quinoa Breakfast Salad 33

Brown Rice And Coconut Bowl 35

Simple Tapioca Pudding 36

Chickpeas And Beans Breakfast Mix 37

Glazed Pork Chops 39

Panini Chicken 40

Penne Pasta 42

Turkey Sandwich 44

Mint Salad 45

Waldorf Salad 46

Chicken & Bacon Salad 47

Grilled Watermelon Steak Salad 48

Crispy Cod And Green Beans 50

Pistachio-Crusted Fish 52

Cumin-Spiced Lamb And Salad 54

Sugar Snap Pea And Radish Salad 56

Horseradish Salmon Cakes 58

Salmon, Green Beans, And Tomatoes 60

Broccoli Pesto Fusilli 62

Strawberry Spinach Salad 64

One-Pot Shrimp And Spinach 65

Spicy Southwestern Rice Bowl 67

Pita Cheese And Veggie Pizza 69

Mushroom And Spinach Mozzarella Wraps 71

Grilled Tofu And Vegetable Salad 73

Stuffed Bell Peppers 75

Scallions Omelet 77

Breakfast Almond Smoothie 78

Fruits And Rice Pudding 79

Asparagus Omelet 80

Bean Frittata 81

Plums And Prunes Oatmeal 82

Tomato Lentils With Arugula And Feta Cheese 83

Tuna Spaghetti 85

Spinach Omelet 87

Vegetable Chicken Pockets 89

Creamy Lime Fruit Salad 89

Citrus Salad... 92

Spaghetti Squash.. 94

Tuna With Vegetables 96

Mix Vegetable Curry With Boil Rice 97

Poached Whitefish 99

Chicken And Broccoli Stir Fry With Brown Rice 100

Chicken And Wild Rice Stuffed Tomatoes................ 102

Fish Tacos 104

Strawberry And Banana Smoothie........................... 106

Shrimp And Artichoke Frittata 107

Easy Spinach And Quinoa Pancakes......................... 109

Orange Yogurt 111

Easy Shrimp Salad 112

Chicken With Noodles.. 114

Chili Con Carne 116

Chili Beans And Sweet Potato 118

Slow Cooker Chicken Soup 120

Chicken Cacciatore 121

Chicken And Wide Rice Stuffed Tomatoes 123

Apple-Cinnamon Granola 125

Beef Stroganoff 127

Baking Apple 129

The Healthy French Toast 131

Oat Pancakes 132

Burrito 134

Ravioli Skillet Lasagna 136

Orange Roast Chicken 138

Salmon With Broccoli & Red Potatoes 140

Whole Grain Pasta & Pumpkin Bake 143

Daphne Oz's Philly Cheesesteak Tacos 145

Vegetables And Turkey Stir-Fry 148

Pantry Minestrone 150

Tex-Mex Loaded Baked Sweet Potatoes 152

Tandoori Chicken 155

Turkey Fajitas Bowls... 157

Sesame-Honey Chicken & Quinoa Bowl................... 159

Southwest Tortilla Bake 162

Flank Steak And Roasted Corn Salad With Vinaigrette 164

Chicken Salad Grilled With Buttermilk Dressing 168

Chicken Burritos 172

Brussels Sprouts With Lemon And Shallots 175

Barley And Tomato Roast Risotto 177

Chia Pudding 181

Chicken Vegetable Bake... 182

Onion Omelette 185

Olive Omelette 186

Tomato Omelette... 187

Tuscan-Style Tuna Salad

Ingredients:

- 3   tablespoons of olive oil extra-virgin
- 3   tablespoons of lemon juice
- scallions trimmed & sliced
- Freshly ground pepper for taste
- 25 to 120 ounce can of small white beans like cannellini/great northern rinsed
- 1/2 teaspoon salt
- 12   cherry tomatoes quartered
- ounce cans of chunk light tuna drained

Directions:

1   In a medium dish, combine the fish, beans, onions, oil, scallions, lemon juice, pepper, and salt.
2   Stir it slowly. Refrigerate until it is ready.

Strawberry, Melon & Avocado Salad

Ingredients:

- tablespoons fresh mint finely chopped
- tablespoons of sherry vinegar/red-wine vinegar
- teaspoons toasted sesame seeds
- cups of baby spinach
- Pinch of salt
- 1 1 cups sliced hulled strawberries
- 1 small avocado 4-5 ounces peeled up, pitted and cut into 17 slices
- 1/2 cup honey
- 1/2 teaspoon ground pepper fresh
- 17 slices of about 1 small cantaloupe thin & rind removed

Directions:

1. In a small cup, whisk the honey, mint, vinegar, pepper and salt.
2. . Divide the Spinach into 4 plates of lettuce.
3. On top of the Spinach, place alternating pieces of cantaloupe and avocado. Top the strawberries for each salad, sprinkle with dressing and scatter with the sesame seeds.

Roast Chicken Dal

Ingredients:

- 1 3 -pound of roasted chicken with discarded skin, meat separated from bones & diced 4 cups
- 1 small onion minced
- ½ cup plain yogurt low-fat
- ½ teaspoon salt for taste
- teaspoons of curry powder
- 1 1 teaspoons of canola oil
- 112 -ounce canned tomatoes diced & preferably fire-roasted
- 112 -ounce lentil Can rinsed or 3 cups of cooked lentils

Directions:

1 Heat oil over medium to high heat heavy saucepan. Include the onion and fry, stirring

for 5 to 4 minutes, until tender but not browned.

2 Add the curry powder and simmer for 3 0 to 5 0 seconds, stirring until mixed with the onion and deep aromatics.

3 Whisk in lentils, tomatoes, salt and chicken and cook until it is heated fully, stirring regularly.

4 Turn off the heat and apply the yogurt, and stir. Serve it instantly.

Spaghetti Squash With Chunky Tomato Sauce

Ingredients:

- cup 1 small green sweet pepper chopped
- 1 teaspoons crushed Italian seasoning dried
- 1/2 cup 1.5 ounce Parmesan cheese shredded
- 1 12 -ounce tomato sauce Can
- teaspoon of black pepper
- 1 pound of lean ground beef
- cloves of minced garlic
- tablespoons of tomato paste
- 1 recipe Cooked Spaghetti Squash
- Small & fresh basil leaves
- 15 ounce Canned tomatoes diced & undrained
- cup 1 medium onion chopped

Directions:

1. Cook the ground beef, sweet pepper onion, and garlic in a wide saucepan until the meat is brown. Drain it. Add the diced and undrained tomatoes, black pepper tomato sauce, tomato paste, and Italian seasoning. Boil the sauce and minimize the heat.
2. Simmer and uncovered for 20 to 26 minutes and stir for some time.
3. . Meanwhile, cooking of the Spaghetti Squash. Serve the sauce over squash. Sprinkle the cheese with Parmesan. Garnish with basil leaves if needed.
4. Cooked Spaghetti Squash: In many spots, a sharp knife pokes a 2 -3 - 5 -pound whole spaghetti squash. Put the squash in a microwave-safe baking dish. Microwave the uncovered for 12 to 20 to 25 minutes on 12 0 percent high capacity or until tender. Let wait for five minutes. Halve the thickness of

the squash and cut the seeds. Shred and split the squash pulp into strands using two forks. Make 7 parts for serving.

Meatier Meatloaf

Ingredients:

- tablespoon of dried thyme
- slice of white sandwich bread split into 1 piece
- cup of ketchup
- 1 tablespoon of hot sauce
- 1 tablespoon of unflavored gelatin
- 1 tablespoon of tomato paste
- 1 onion chopped & fine
- 1-pound ground pork
- 1-pound lean ground beef 12   5%
- 7   oz. of white mushrooms trimmed & thinly sliced
- 4 pepper
- 5   tablespoons with 1   cup chicken broth low-sodium

- tablespoons of packed brown sugar
- tablespoons of Dijon mustard
- 1 tablespoons of unsalted butter
- tablespoons of soy sauce
- 1 large eggs
- minced garlic cloves
- 1/2 cup of cider vinegar
- 1/10 cup fresh parsley minced
- tablespoon of ground coriander

Directions:

1. For the meatloaf: Change the oven rack's center location and fire the oven to 5 50 degrees Fahrenheit.
2. Fold heavy-duty aluminum foil into a 5-inch rectangle to form 9. Cover the foil in a rimmed baking sheet mounted on a wire shelf.

3   Poke holes with a skewer approximately 1 inch apart in the foil. Spray the foil with a spray of vegetable oil.

4   . In a 15 inch skillet over medium heat, melt the butter. Add the onion and mushrooms; fry and stirring regularly for 12 to 15 minutes, until the color is brown.

5   Add the tomato paste and simmer for about 5 minutes and mix continuously, until browned.

6   Reduce heat to low and add 5 tablespoons of broth and garlic. Cook to remove any browned pieces, scraping the plate's bottom until thickened, for around 1 minute.

7   To cool, shift the mushroom mixture to a wide dish.

5   Whisk together the eggs, the remaining half a cup of broth, and the soy sauce in a bowl. Sprinkle the gelatin over the egg mixture and leave to rest for about 5 minutes until the gelatin softens.

8   Pulse the bread until finely ground in the food processor at 5 to 12   pulses.
9   To bread-crumbs, add gelatin blend, cooled mushroom blend, mustard, parsley, thyme and pepper.
10 And pulse them until the mushrooms are finely ground, around 12   pulses, scraping down the bowl as desired. Place the bread-crumb mixture in a wide dish.
11 To fully blend, add pork and beef and meld with your hands.
12 Move the meat mixture to the rectangle foil and use wet hands to create a 9 by 5-inch loaf.
13 Bake the meatloaf for 75 to 90 minutes until the heat reaches 20 to 25 5 to 17   0 degrees Fahrenheit. Take the broiler from the oven and turn it on.
14 For the glaze: When the meatloaf is frying, put all the Ingredients: in a small saucepan

over medium heat to boil. Cook and stirring regularly for about 5 minutes, until it becomes thick and syrupy.

15 Spread half of the glaze uniformly over the cooked meatloaf; put under the broiler and cook for around 3 minutes before the glaze bubbles and starts browning at the edges. Remove the meatloaf from the oven and cover thinly with the remaining glaze. Return to the broiler and cook for about 3 minutes longer before the glaze bursts again and starts to brown. Before slicing and serving, let the meatloaf cool for 30 minutes.

Pork Tenderloin Curry In Apple Cider

Ingredients:

- Olive oil extra-virgin 1 tablespoon
- Yellow onions chopped 3   medium
- Apple cider 3   cups
- Tart apple 1
- Cornstarch 1 tablespoon
- Pork tenderloin 17   ounces
- Curry powder 1 ½ tablespoons

Directions:

1   Begin by cutting the pork tenderloin into 4 equal-sized pieces.
2   Take the tart apple; peel and remove the seeds. Cut the apple into bite-sized chunks.
3   Take a shallow dish and place the pork tenderloin into the same. Sprinkle the tenderloin pieces with curry powder and use

your hands to coat the meat evenly. Set aside for around 20 to 25 minutes.

4. Take a cast-iron skillet and place it on a medium-high flame. Pour in the olive oil and let it heat through.
5. Add the pork tenderloin pieces to the skillet and cook for 7 minutes; flip over and cook for another 7 minutes.
6. Once done, put the pork onto a plate and set it aside.
7. Return the skillet to the flame and toss in the onions. Once the onions begin to caramelize, add the 1 ½ cups of apple cider. Reduce the flame and let the sauce simmer until it reduces to half.
8. Now add in the chopped tart apple, ½ cup of apple cider, and cornstarch. Give it a nice stir and let it simmer for about 3 minutes or until the sauce thickens.

9 Return the pork tenderloins to the sauce and cook for another 5 minutes on a low flame.
10 Once done, use a tong to place the pork tenderloins on a serving platter. Pour the prepared sauce over the meat.
11 Serve and enjoy!

Clams Fettuccine

Ingredients:

- Corn kernels 3   cups
- White wine ½ cup
- Olive oil 1 tablespoon
- Fresh basil chopped 4 tablespoons
- Clams drained 3   cans
- Salt ¼ teaspoon
- Black pepper freshly ground as per taste
- Fettuccine uncooked 12   ounces
- Garlic minced 3   tablespoons
- Tomatoes 3   large

Directions:

1. Begin by seeding the tomatoes and cutting them into small chunks. Set aside.
2. Take a large stockpot and fill it halfway with water. Let it come to a boil.

3. Throw in the pasta and cook for around 12 minutes. Once done, drain it into a colander and set aside.
4. Take a large nonstick saucepan and add in the olive oil, garlic, corn, tomatoes, basil, and wine. Mix well and cover the pan with a lid. Keep stirring and let it come to a boil.
5. Once the sauce comes to a boil, reduce the flame and toss in the clams and cooked fettuccine.
6. Season the pasta with pepper and salt. Mix well.
7. Serve immediately.

Strip Steak With Mushroom Whiskey Sauce

Ingredients:

- Shiitake mushrooms sliced 3 ounces
- Button mushrooms 3 ounces
- Thyme ¼ teaspoon
- Rosemary ¼ teaspoon
- Whiskey ¼ cup
- New York strip steaks 3
- Margarine trans-free 1 teaspoon
- Garlic chopped 5 cloves

Directions:

1. Begin by preparing a fire in the charcoal grill.
2. Take the grill rack and coat it lightly with cooking spray. Place the grill rack about 7 inches above the fire.

3. Place the steak onto the grill and cook for around 12 minutes; flip over and cook for another 12 minutes.
4. Take a nonstick saucepan and place it on a medium flame. Add in the margarine and let it heat through. Add in the garlic, thyme, rosemary, and mushrooms. Sauté for around 3 minutes or until the mushrooms are tender.
5. Once done, remove the saucepan from the flame and pour in the whiskey. Cook for about a minute.
6. Place the steaks on a serving plate and top them with the whiskey sautéed mushrooms. Serve and enjoy!

Creamy Polenta With Veggies

Ingredients:

- Fresh mushrooms sliced 1 cup
- Onions sliced 1 cup
- Broccoli florets 1 cup
- Zucchini sliced 1 cup
- Parmesan cheese grated 3 tablespoons
- Fresh oregano chopped as per taste
- Cornmeal/polenta coarsely ground 1 cup
- Water 4 cups
- Garlic chopped 1 teaspoon

Directions:

1. Begin by preheating the oven by setting the temperature to 5 50 degrees Fahrenheit.
2. Take a glass baking dish and lightly coat it with cooking spray.

3. Add polenta, garlic, and water to a mixing bowl and mix well. Transfer into the baking dish.
4. Place the baking dish into the oven and bake for around 40 minutes.
5. While the polenta cooks, place the nonstick pan on a medium flame. Coat the pan with cooking spray.
6. Once the pan is hot, add in the onions and mushrooms. Sauté until the veggies are nicely tender; this will take around 5 minutes.
7. Place a steamer on a medium-high flame and add the zucchini and broccoli to the steamer basket. Cover the lid and steam for around 5 minutes. The veggies should be tender yet crisp.
8. Once the polenta is done, take the baking dish out of the oven and top it with steamed zucchini and broccoli.

9   Finish by sprinkling the veggies with herbs and parmesan cheese.
10 Serve right away!

Chicken Salad With Balsamic Vinaigrette And Pineapple

Ingredients:

- Broccoli florets 3 cups
- Fresh baby spinach 4 cups
- Red onions thinly sliced ½ cup
- Chicken breasts boneless and skinless 4
- Olive oil 1 tablespoon
- Pineapple chunks unsweetened 1 12 -ounce can save 3 tablespoons of juice

For Vinaigrette:

- Sugar 3 teaspoons
- Cinnamon ground ¼ teaspoon
- Olive oil ¼ cup
- Balsamic vinegar 3 tablespoons

Directions:

1. Begin by cutting the chicken breasts into bite-sized cubes.
2. Take a large nonstick pan and place it on a medium flame. Pour in the olive oil and let it heat through.
3. Once the oil is hot, add in the chicken and sauté for around 12 minutes. Make sure the chicken is golden brown and slightly charred on the edges.
4. Take a large glass mixing bowl and add in the pineapple chunks, spinach, broccoli, onions, and chicken chunks. Toss well and set aside
5. To prepare the dressing, add the olive oil, reserved pineapple juice, vinegar, cinnamon, and sugar to a glass mixing bowl. Mix well to combine.
6. Pour the prepared dressing onto the chicken and veggies and toss until all Ingredients: are evenly coated.

7. Transfer onto a salad platter and serve!

Mushroom Oatmeal

Ingredients:

- ½ cup fat-free cheese, grated
- ounces mushroom, sliced
- 15   ounces low-sodium chicken stock
- 1 small yellow onion, chopped
- 1 cup old-fashioned rolled oats
- thyme springs, chopped
- garlic cloves, minced
- tablespoons olive oil
- 1 Black pepper to the taste
- ½ cup water

Directions:

1   Set your instant pot on sauté mode, add the oil, heat it up, add onions and garlic, stir, cook for 4 minutes, add oats, water, pepper, stock

and thyme, cover and cook at High for 12 minutes.

2 Add mushrooms, stir, cover the pot, cook on High for 5 minutes more, divide into bowls, sprinkle the cheese on top and serve for breakfast.

Eggs Mix

Ingredients:

- eggs
- 1 and 1/10 cup water
- scallions, chopped
- A pinch of black pepper
- ½ teaspoon garlic powder
- ½ teaspoon sesame seeds

Directions:

1. In a bowl, mix the eggs with 1/10 cup water, whisk well, strain into a baking dish that fits your instant pot, add black pepper, garlic powder, sesame seeds and scallions and whisk.
2. Add the rest of the water to your instant pot, add steamer basket, add baking dish inside, cover, cook on High for 5 minutes, divide between plates and serve.

Carrot Oatmeal

Ingredients:

- tablespoons maple syrup
- 1 teaspoon pumpkin pie spice
- cups water
- ¼ cup chia seeds
- 1 cup steel cut oats
- 1 cup carrots, grated
- 1 tablespoon fat-free butter
- teaspoons cinnamon powder

Directions:

1 Set your instant pot on sauté mode, add the butter, heat it up, add oats and cook them for 5   minutes.
2   Add carrots, water, maple syrup, cinnamon and spice, cover the pot and cook on High for

12 minutes. Add chia seeds, stir, divide into bowls and serve for breakfast.

Dates And Millet Pudding

Ingredients:

- 1 cup millet
- ounces water
- dates, pitted
- 20 to 25   ounces coconut milk

Directions:

1   Put the millet in your instant pot, add dates, milk and water, stir, cover, cook on High for 12   minutes, divide into bowls and serve for breakfast.

Quinoa Breakfast Salad

Ingredients:

- 1 jalapeno pepper, chopped
- ½ cup scallions, chopped
- 1 and ½ cups canned chickpeas, no-salt-added, drained
- 1/10 cup mint, chopped
- tablespoons veggie stock
- and ¼ cups water
- ¼ cup lime juice
- Black pepper to the taste
- garlic cloves, minced
- 1 avocado, pitted, peeled and diced
- tomatoes, chopped
- 1 and ½ cups quinoa, rinsed
- 1 cucumber, chopped

- 3 /5   cup parsley, chopped

Directions:

1   In your instant pot, mix quinoa with half of the garlic and the water, stir, cover, cook on High for 4 minutes, fluff with a fork, transfer to a bowl, add tomatoes, cucumber, jalapeno, scallions, chickpeas, parsley, mint and avocado and toss.

2   In a bowl, mix the stock with black pepper, the rest of the garlic and lime juice, whisk, add to salad, toss and serve for breakfast.

Brown Rice And Coconut Bowl

Ingredients:

- ¼ cup almonds
- ¼ cup raisins
- 1 cup water
- A pinch of cinnamon powder
- 1 cup coconut milk
- 1 cup brown rice
- ½ cup maple syrup

Directions:

1. In your instant pot, mix the rice with the water, milk, almonds, raisins, cinnamon and maple syrup, stir well, cover the pot, cook on High for 20 to 25 minutes, divide into bowls and serve for breakfast.

Simple Tapioca Pudding

Ingredients:

- 1/10 cup tapioca pearls
- tablespoons coconut sugar
- Zest of ½ lemon, grated
- 1 and ¼ cup low-fat milk
- 1 and ½ cups water

Directions:

1. Put tapioca in a heatproof bowl, add milk, ½ cup water, lemon zest and sugar and toss.
2. Add the water to your instant pot, add the steamer basket, add the bowl inside, cover, cook on High for 12 minutes, divide into bowls and serve.

Chickpeas And Beans Breakfast Mix

Ingredients:

- tablespoons apple cider vinegar
- 1 cup cranberry beans, soaked and drained
- ½ red onion, chopped
- 1 garlic clove, minced
- 1 and ½ cups green beans
- celery stalks, chopped
- A pinch of black pepper
- 1 bay leaf
- 1 cup chickpeas, soaked and drained
- tablespoons olive oil

Directions:

1. In your instant pot, mix the water with chickpeas, bay leaf and garlic and stir.
2. Add steamer basket, add cranberry and green beans inside, cover, cook on High for 20 to 25

minutes, drain everything and transfer them to a salad bowl.

3. Add celery, onion, vinegar, oil and pepper, toss well and serve for breakfast.

Glazed Pork Chops

Ingredients:

- tablespoons water
- 1 cup all-purpose flour
- pork loin chops
- ½ cup maple syrup
- 1 tablespoon cornstarch
- 1 cup brown sugar
- pinch of salt

Directions:

- In a bowl combine salt and flour together
- Place the pork chops in the bowl and turn to coat
- Place pork chops in a skillet and cook until golden brown
- Add maple syrup, sugar, water cornstarch, and bring to a boil

- Cook until the sugar is dissolved and meat is cooked
- When ready remove from the skillet and serve

Panini Chicken

Ingredients:

- ½ cup chicken broth
- ¼ tsp salt
- ¼ tsp turmeric
- green onion
- 1 lb. chicken breast
- 1 tsp gingerroot

Directions:

1. In a slow cooker place your chicken and add broth, garlic clove, green onions and gingerroot
2. When ready remove chicken mixture and place the chicken on a flatbread

3. Cook sandwich in a panini maker
4. When ready remove and serve

Penne Pasta

Ingredients:

- 1 tablespoon basil
- ¼ cup white wine
- 1 tablespoon tomato paste
- 1 tablespoon all-purpose flour
- 1 cup parmesan cheese
- 1 package penne pasta
- 1 onion
- 1 tablespoon thyme

Directions:

1. In a stockpot cook pasta al dente
2. In a skillet sauté onion until soft, add salt, herbs, tomato paste, flour and cook for 3 -5 minutes
3. Add pasta to the tomato mixture and bring to a boil

4 When ready serve with parmesan cheese on top

Turkey Sandwich

Ingredients:

- 1 loaf bread
- Lettuce
- 1 lb. cooked turkey
- ½ lb. swiss cheese
- 1 tomato
- oz. cream cheese
- tablespoons salad dressing
- 1 tsp garlic powder

Directions:

1. In a bowl combine cream cheese, garlic powder and salad dressing
2. Spread mixture on the bread
3. Add lettuce, tomatoes, cheese and turkey
4. Serve when ready

Mint Salad

Ingredients:

- Mint leaves
- spring onions
- tablespoons olive oil
- tablespoons lemon juice
- 1 lb. broad beans
- ½ lb. peas
- chives

Directions:

1. In a bowl combine all Ingredients: together and mix well
2. . Serve with dressing

Waldorf Salad

Ingredients:

- 1 cup apples
- 1 cup celery
- ¼ cup parsley
- 1 cup walnuts
- 1 tablespoon mayonnaise
- 1 tablespoon Greek Yogurt
- 1 cup grapes
- 1 cup lettuce

Directions:

1. In a bowl combine all Ingredients: together and mix well
2. Serve with dressing

Chicken & Bacon Salad

Ingredients:

- ½ cup cooked bacon
- 1 tablespoon chives
- ½ cup salad dressing
- 1 lb. penne
- 1 tablespoon olive oil
- lb. cooked chicken breasts

Directions:

1 In a bowl combine all Ingredients: together and mix well
2 . Serve with dressing

Grilled Watermelon Steak Salad

Ingredients:

- Onion 1 tsp., small red
- Parsley 1 c., chopped
- Salt and pepper
- Sirloin steak 1 lb.
- Unsalted peanuts to garnish
- Watermelon 5 lbs., seedless
- Cherry tomatoes 1 lb., halved
- Honey 1 tsp
- Lemon juice 5 Tbsp.
- Mint leaves 1 c., torn up
- Olive oil 3 Tbsp.

Directions:

1. Prepare grill to medium-high. Season steak, then grill until done to preference. Allow it to rest on a cutting board.

2. Mix oil, lemon juice, honey, and seasonings. Incorporate the onions and tomatoes as well, folding in nicely.
3. Cut watermelon into 0.5-inch thick triangles and remove rinds. Oil and grill until starting to char—a minute per side, then set aside.
4. Mix the herbs into the tomato mixture. Serve with watermelon topped with stead.

Crispy Cod And Green Beans

Ingredients:

- Pepper to taste
- Pesto 3 Tbsp.
- Salt to taste
- Skinless cod 1.3 5 lb., four pieces
- Green Beans 1 lb.
- Olive oil 3 Tbsp.
- Parmesan cheese 0.3 5 c., grated

Directions:

1. Set oven to 43 5 F. Put beans onto rimmed baking sheet and combine with 1 Tbsp. oil, then top with cheese and a sprinkling of seasonings. Roast for 12 -15 minutes, waiting for it to finally start to brown.

2. Heat remaining oil in a skillet. Season cod and cook until golden brown. You want to use a medium-high heat to do this.
3. Serve with pesto over cod, next to a bed of green beans.

Pistachio-Crusted Fish

Ingredients:

- Pepper 0.5 tsp
- Quinoa 0.75 c.
- Salt 0.75 tsp
- Shelled pistachios, chopped 0.3 5 c.
- Tilapia 4 7 -oz. pieces
- Baby spinach 4 c.
- Greek yogurt 4 Tbsp.
- Lemon juice 3 Tbsp.
- Olive oil 3 Tbsp.
- Panko whole-wheat, 0.3 5 c.

Directions:

1. Prepare quinoa based on instructions on packaging.
2. Season fish with salt, pepper, and coat with 1 Tbsp. each of Greek yogurt.

3. Combine panko and pistachios, tossing with 1 Tbsp. olive oil. Gently sprinkle over the top of the fish, pressing it to stick. Bake for 15 minutes at 5 75 F., or until done.
4. Combine cooked quinoa with spinach, lemon juice, remaining oil, and a pinch of salt and pepper. Serve with fish.

Cumin-Spiced Lamb And Salad

Ingredients:

- Salt and pepper to taste
- Carrots 1 lb.
- Cumin 1.3 5 tsp.
- Honey 0.5 tsp.
- Lamb loin chops 12 —about 3 lbs.
- Mint leaves 0.3 5 c., fresh
- Olive oil 5   Tbsp.
- Radishes 7
- Red wine vinegar 3   Tbsp.

Directions:

1. Combine 3   Tbsp. oil, vinegar, a pinch of cumin, honey, and salt and pepper.
2. Warm remaining oil in a skillet at medium. Season lamb with cumin and a pinch of salt and pepper. Cook until preferred doneness.

3. Shave carrots into pieces and create thinly sliced radishes. Coat with dressing and mix with mint. Serve with lamb.

Sugar Snap Pea And Radish Salad

Ingredients:

- Ground coriander 0.3 5 tsp
- Olive oil 0.3 5 c.
- Radishes 15 , small
- Salt o.5 tsp
- Sugar snap peas 1 lb.
- Watermelon radish 1, small
- Apple-cider vinegar 3 Tbsp.
- Avocado 0.5, medium ripe
- Dijon mustard 0.5 tsp
- Fresh lemon juice 1 Tbsp.
- Freshly ground pepper 0.5 tsp

Directions:

1. Combine peas and radishes in a bowl together.

2. In a blender, combine everything else and puree until well combined and smooth. Add water if necessary to thin it out.
3. Coat radish and peas with dressing and serve.

Horseradish Salmon Cakes

Ingredients:

- Olive oil 3   Tbsp.
- Panko 0.3 5 c.
- Salt and pepper to taste
- Skinless salmon filet 1.3 5 lb.
- Watercress 1 bunch
- Dijon mustard 1 Tbsp.
- English cucumber 1, small
- Greek Yogurt 3   Tbsp.
- Horseradish 3   Tbsp.
- Lemon juice 1 Tbsp.

Directions:

1. Combine salmon, horseradish, salt and pepper, and mustard into a food processor until well chopped. Then, toss in the bread crumbs and combine well.

2. Form 12 patties.
3. Warm 1 Tbsp. oil in a skillet. Cook until opaque throughout, typically 3 minutes before flipping.
4. Combine yogurt, lemon juice, oil, and a sprinkle of salt and pepper. Combine in cucumber slices, then watercress.
5. Serve salmon with salad.

Salmon, Green Beans, And Tomatoes

Ingredients:

- Anchovy fillets 5
- Olive oil 3 Tbsp.
- Kosher salt and pepper to personal preference
- Salmon fillet, skinless
- Garlic 7 cloves
- Green beans 1 lb.
- Grape tomatoes 1 pint
- Kalamata olives 0.5 c.

Directions:

1. Prepare oven to 43 5 F. Put beans, garlic, olive, anchovy, and tomatoes together along with half of the oil and a pinch of pepper. Roast until veggies are tender.

2. Warm the remainder of the oil over a skillet at medium heat. Season salmon, then cook until done. Serve salmon and veggies together.

Broccoli Pesto Fusilli

Ingredients:

- Lemon zest 1 Tbsp.
- Olive oil 5   Tbsp.
- Parmesan cheese to garnish
- Salt to taste
- Sliced almonds to garnish
- Basil leaves 0.5 c.
- Broccoli florets 15   oz.
- Fusilli 15   oz.
- Garlic 3   cloves

Directions:

1. Prepare pasta to directions and reserve 0.5 c. of the liquid.
2. Combine broccoli, garlic, and the reserved water in a bowl and cook for five or six minutes, stirring halfway through. Put everything right into a food processor with

the liquid. Combine in basil, oil, zest, a pinch of salt, and puree.

3. Put pasta in with pesto. Drizzle in water if necessary. Sprinkle with cheese and nuts if desired. Serve immediately.

Strawberry Spinach Salad

Ingredients:

- Sliced strawberries 0.5 c.
- Vinaigrette of choice 3 Tbsp.
- Walnut pieces roasted
- Baby spinach 5 c.
- Medium avocado 0.3 5, diced
- Red onion 1 Tbsp.

Directions:

1. Combine spinach with the berries and onion.
2. Mix well. Coat with vinaigrette and toss.
3. Then, top with walnuts and avocado. Serve.

One-Pot Shrimp And Spinach

Ingredients:

- Olive oil 5 Tbsp.
- Parsley 1 Tbsp.
- Salt to personal preference
- Shrimp 1 lb.
- Spinach 1 lb.
- Crushed red pepper 0.3 5 tsp
- Garlic 7 cloves, sliced
- Lemon juice 1 Tbsp.
- Lemon zest 1.5 tsp.

Directions:

1. Warm skillet with 1 Tbsp.
2. oil. Cook half of the garlic until browning, about a single minute.
3. Then, toss in spinach and salt. Wait for it to wilt over the heat, about 5 minutes.

4. Remove and mix in lemon juice, storing it in a separate bowl.
5. Warm heat to medium-high and toss with remainder of oil.
6. Toss in the rest of your garlic and cook until browning.
7. Then, mix in shrimp, pepper, and salt.
8. Cook until shrimp is done, then serve atop spinach with lemon zest and parsley garnish.

Spicy Southwestern Rice Bowl

Ingredients:

- Tomato 1
- Zucchini 1
- Vegetable Oil 1 t.
- Low-fat Cheese 3 T.
- Low-fat Sour Cream 3 T.
- Salsa 4 T.
- Brown Rice, Cooked 1 C.
- Lean Meat, Cooked 1 C.
- Bell Peppers 1
- Onion 1
- Corn 1 Can

Directions:

1 To begin, prepare all of the vegetables from the list above. Be sure to clean and peel before you begin cooking.
2 Once they are ready, take a medium skillet over medium heat and cook all of the vegetables for around five minutes. Once they are done, the vegetables should be soft.
3 Now that your veggies are cooked, go ahead and toss in the cooked lean meat and the cooked rice.
4 Mix everything together and then portion it into four bowls.
5 If desired, top everything with cheese, sour cream, and salsa for extra flavor.

Pita Cheese And Veggie Pizza

Ingredients:

- Tomato Sauce .3 5 C.
- Mozzarella Cheese .50 C.
- Whole Wheat Pita Bread 3   Pieces
- Mushrooms .50 C.
- Bell Pepper 1
- Onion 1

Directions:

1. You will start by heating your oven to 5   50 degrees.
2. While this heats up, separate the pita pockets and spoon in your vegetables, cheese, and tomato sauce.
3. Once the pita pockets are prepared, you will want to wrap them up into aluminum foil and bake them for around ten minutes.

4. When the cheese is nice and melted, remove from the oven, allow to cool and your lunch will be ready to serve.

Mushroom And Spinach Mozzarella Wraps

Ingredients:

- Garlic 1 T.
- Mushrooms 1 C.
- Olive Oil 1 T.
- Whole Wheat Wraps 3
- Low-Fat Mozzarella .3 5 C.
- Tomato 1
- Spinach 1 C.

Directions:

1. Begin by heating your oven to 5 50 degrees.
2. While this warms up, take a medium pan over medium heat and place your one tablespoon of olive oil. When the olive oil begins to sizzle, place the garlic and mushrooms and sauté them for about five minutes.

3. On your wraps, begin to layer the tomato, spinach, cooked mushrooms, and mozzarella cheese.
4. Carefully wrap all of the Ingredients: and place them into a baking dish.
5. Place the wraps in your oven for about ten minutes and remove once the cheese has melted.
6. Cut your wraps in half, allow them to cool, and serve warm!

Grilled Tofu And Vegetable Salad

Ingredients:

- Red Pepper 3
- Summer Squash 1
- Reduced-Fat Tofu 1 Lb.
- Low-fat Italian Salad Dressing .75 C.
- Spinach 1 C.
- Barley .50 C.
- Quinoa .50 C.

Directions:

1. Please note that before you begin this recipe, we suggest you prepare your tofu the night before. You can do this by slicing the tofu into slices and soaking in the Italian salad dressing. Once the tofu is drenched, add in your prepared vegetables and allow all of the Ingredients: to soak for twenty-four hours.

2. The next day, drain the tofu and vegetables of any excess liquids. Place the Ingredients: into a medium size pan over medium heat and cook for about eight minutes on each side.
3. By the end, the tofu and vegetables should be crispy and then removed from the heat.
4. When your tofu and vegetables are cooked, you will want to cook your quinoa according to the package directions. This normally takes around fifteen minutes or so. If desired, also add in the barley to your quinoa and be sure it is all cooked through.
5. Now, toss all of the Ingredients: into a large bowl and mix everything together.
6. Once this is done, your salad is ready to be served. It makes an excellent side dish or a light lunch.

Stuffed Bell Peppers

Ingredients:

- Cayenne Pepper .20 To 25 T.
- Chili Powder 1 T.
- Cumin 1 T.
- Black Beans 1 Can
- Salsa 1.50 C.
- Bell Peppers 4
- Frozen Corn 1.50 C.
- Brown Rice .50 C.
- Low-Fat Cheese .50 C.

Directions:

1. You can start off by cooking the brown rice according to the directions on the box.
2. As the rice cooks, begin to prepare your peppers by slicing them in half and removing the seeds.

3. Next, place the peppers on a greased baking dish and broil them for five minutes on each side in your oven.
4. As the peppers cook, prepare your bean mixture. Take a small mixing bowl and add in the spices, salsa, beans, corn, and part of the cheese.
5. Pop the bowl into the microwave for three minutes and stir everything together.
6. Once the cheese has melted, you can spoon this mixture into your cooked peppers. Sprinkle the cheese on top and broil for another two minutes.
7. Remove the peppers from the oven, allow to cool, then serve warm!

Scallions Omelet

Ingredients:

- 1 tablespoon low-fat low-fat sour cream
- ¼ teaspoon ground black pepper
- 1 teaspoon olive oil
- 1 oz scallions, chopped
- eggs, beaten

Directions:

1. Heat up olive oil in the skillet.
2. meanwhile, in the mixing bowl mix up all remaining Ingredients:
3. pour the egg mixture in the hot skillet, flatten well and cook for 7 minutes over the medium-low heat.
4. the omelet is cooked when it is set.

Breakfast Almond Smoothie

Ingredients:

- ½ cup almonds, chopped
- 1 cup low-fat milk
- 1 banana, peeled, chopped

Directions:

1. Put all ingredients: in the blender and blend until smooth.
2. pour the smoothie in the serving glasses.

Fruits And Rice Pudding

Ingredients:

- 1 teaspoon vanilla extract
- oz apricots, chopped
- ½ cup long-grain rice
- 1 ½ cup low-fat milk

Directions:

1. Pour milk and add rice in the saucepan.
2. Close the lid and cook the rice on the medium-high heat for 12 minutes.
3. Then add vanilla extract and stir the rice well.
4. Transfer the pudding in the bowls and top

Asparagus Omelet

Ingredients:

- eggs, beaten
- tablespoons low-fat milk
- 1 teaspoon avocado oil
- oz asparagus, boiled, chopped
- ¼ teaspoon ground paprika
- ½ teaspoon ground cumin

Directions:

1. Heat up avocado oil in the skillet.
2. Meanwhile, mix up ground paprika, ground cumin. Eggs, and milk.
3. Pour the liquid in the hot skillet and cook it for 3 minutes.
4. Then add chopped asparagus and close the lid.
5. Cook the omelet for 5 minutes on low heat.

Bean Frittata

Ingredients:

- ½ onion, diced
- 1 tablespoon margarine
- 1 teaspoon dried dill
- eggs, beaten
- ½ cup red kidney beans, canned

Directions:

1. toss the margarine in the skillet. Add onion and saute it for 4 minutes or until it is soft.
2. then add red kidney beans and dried dill. Mix the mixture up.
3. pour the eggs over it and close the lid.
4. cook the frittata on medium-low heat for 7 minutes or until it is set or bake it in the oven at 5　90f for 5 minutes.

Plums And Prunes Oatmeal

Ingredients:

- 1 diced fresh plums
- ¼ cup diced prunes
- 1 tablespoon maple syrup
- A dash or two of cinnamon
- ¾ cup old fashioned rolled oats
- ¾ cup fat-free milk
- ¼ cup apple cider

Directions:

1. Heat milk in a saucepan, stirring constantly,
2. Cook the oatmeal for 12 minutes or until bubbling and thickened.
3. Add the apple cider, plums and prunes.
4. Add the maple syrup. Sprinkle with a dash or two of cinnamon.

Tomato Lentils With Arugula And Feta Cheese

Ingredients:

- scooped out big tomatoes
- 1 ounce crumbled feta cheese
- 1 cup chopped arugula
- teaspoons dried thyme
- teaspoons vinegar
- ¾ cup whole green lentils
- cups of water
- bay leaves
- 1 teaspoon dried oregano

Directions:

1. Simmer green lentils, water, bay leaves and oregano for about 3 0 minutes or until tender. Drain off cooking liquid.
2. In a mixing bowl, combine lentils, tomatoes, feta cheese, arugula, thyme and vinegar.
3. Stuff the cooked mixture inside the scooped out big tomatoes.
4. Serve.

Tuna Spaghetti

Ingredients:

- 1 cup fresh plum tomatoes
- 1 teaspoon drained and rinsed capers
- 1 cup fresh spinach
- 1 ounces cubed fresh tuna
- ½ tablespoon marjoram
- ounces whole-wheat spaghetti
- ½ diced yellow onion
- ½ teaspoon anchovy paste
- 1 clove minced garlic
- ½ minced chipotle chili

Directions:

1. Sauté onion, garlic, anchovy paste and chipotle chili on a skillet for 3 minutes.
2. Mix in capers and tomatoes, and sauté for two more minutes.

3. Add the spinach and tuna and cook for 90 seconds.
4. Sprinkle the marjoram.
5. Serve the sauce over 3 ounces of cooked whole-wheat spaghetti.

Spinach Omelet

Ingredients:

- eggs
- tablespoons fresh chives
- cups spinach leaves
- ½ cup shredded reduced-fat cheddar cheese
- teaspoon cayenne pepper
- Red pepper relish
- Salt

Directions:

1 Heat a frying pan.
2 Combine eggs and chives in a bowl. Season with salt and cayenne pepper.
3 Whisk the eggs and pour into the frying pan.
4 Stir the eggs and cook for about 5   0 seconds. Sprinkle with cheese. Top with red pepper

relish and spinach. Lift and fold one side of the omelet over the filling.

Vegetable Chicken Pockets

Ingredients

- ¼ cup reduced-fat ranch salad dressing
- ¼ cup shredded carrot
- 1 ½ cups chopped cooked chicken
- ¼ cup chopped broccoli
- 1-inch whole-wheat pita bread rounds
- ¼ cup plain low-fat yogurt
- ¼ cup chopped pecans

Directions:

a. Mix yogurt and ranch salad dressing in a bowl.
b. Combine broccoli, carrot, chicken and pecans in a bowl. Pour yogurt and ranch salad mixture over the chicken and coat well.
c. Spoon the chicken mixture into the whole-wheat pita halves.

Creamy Lime Fruit Salad

Ingredients:

- 1 teaspoons finely shredded lemon peel
- tablespoons powdered sugar
- cups assorted fruits strawberries, kiwi, mango, raspberries, Clementine and pineapple
- tablespoons lime juice

- ½ cup light dairy sour cream
- 1/10 cup fat-free light mayonnaise dressing
- 1 tablespoons lime juice

Directions:

1. Combine sour cream, mayonnaise dressing, sugar, lime juice and lime peel in a mixing bowl.
2. Pour sour cream mixture over the mixed fruits.
3. Day 5

Citrus Salad

Ingredients:

- tablespoons orange juice
- cups spring greens
- 1 tablespoon balsamic vinegar
- tablespoons olive oil
- tablespoons pine nuts
- 1 grapefruit
- oranges

Directions:

1. Slice the oranges and grapefruit and put them in a bowl.
2. In a bowl, combine the olive oil orange juice and vinegar. Pour the dressing over the fruits and coat them well.

3. Place the spring greens on a plate. Before serving, top with the fruit and dressing mixture. Sprinkle with pine nuts.

Spaghetti Squash

Ingredients:

- 1 can of un-drained diced tomatoes
- 3 tablespoons tomato paste
- 1 can of tomato sauce
- ½ teaspoon crushed Italian seasoning
- ¼ cup shredded parmesan cheese
- Black pepper
- 1 cooked spaghetti squash
- 1 pound lean ground beef
- 3 minced garlic cloves
- ½ cup chopped green sweet pepper

Directions:

1. In a pot, combine ground beef, onion, garlic and sweet pepper. Cook until the meat is brown. Mix in un-drained diced tomatoes, tomato paste, and tomato sauce. Season with black pepper and Italian seasoning.

2. Bring the tomato sauce to a boil and simmer for 20 to 25 more minutes.
3. To prepare Spaghetti Squash:
4. Microwave squash for 20 to 25 minutes or until tender.
5. Slice the squash into halves and remove seeds.
6. Shred the squash into strands.
7. Serve the sauce over the spaghetti squash. Sprinkle with parmesan cheese.

Tuna With Vegetables

Ingredients

- tablespoons light mayonnaise
- 1 cup carrots, grated
- Pinch of sea salt
- Pepper to taste
- 1 cup of non-salted tuna, drained
- boiled eggs, diced

Directions

1. Peel the boil eggs and cut lengthwise.
2. Remove the yolk and set aside the whites.
3. In a bowl, mix together tuna, egg yolks, mayonnaise, carrots, salt and pepper.
4. Fill the egg whites with the mixture and garnish with red chilies and olives.
5. Serve .

Mix Vegetable Curry With Boil Rice

Ingredients

- 1 cup broccoli, boiled
- cups cabbage, boiled
- cups carrots. Cubed and boiled
- 1 cup peas, boiled
- boiled beetroots, washed, peeled, coiled
- tablespoons olive oil, for frying
- 1 tablespoon ginger garlic paste
- tablespoons water
- onions, chopped
- 1 teaspoon cumin
- 1 teaspoon red chili flakes
- 1/2 teaspoon cayenne pepper
- 1/2 teaspoon salt
- 1 teaspoon sugar

Directions

1. Boil the rice just before starting the cooking process.
2. Now take a large pan and heat oil in it.
3. Now sauté the onions in the olive oil.
4. Add in ginger garlic paste.
5. Cook for 7 to 8 minutes and then add red chili flakes, cumin, salt, sugar and cayenne pepper.
6. Add in all the boiled vegetables along with water and cook with lid on for about 20 to 25 to 20 minutes.
7. Serve with boiled rice.

Poached Whitefish

Ingredients:

- 1 -1   pounds of whitefish fillets
- 1 pinch saffron
- 3 tablespoons of fennel seeds
- 3 cups of diced tomatoes
- 1 cup of water
- 3 tablespoons of olive oil
- 1 bulbs fennel, chopped
- 3 onion, chopped

Directions:

1 Heat olive oil in a skillet and sauté onion.
2 Add in fennel bulbs and stir.
3 Once onion get soft and tender, add in tomatoes, water and saffron.
4 Add in the fish and fennel seeds at the end, cover the lid and cook for about 20 to 25 minutes. Serve and enjoy.

Chicken And Broccoli Stir Fry With Brown Rice

Ingredients:

- cups of fresh broccoli florets
- 1 cup of snow peas, frozen
- 1 cup of cabbage, shredded
- cups of cooked brown rice
- 1 tablespoon of sesame seed, optional
- 1/10 cup orange juice, freshly squeezed
- 1 tablespoon of low-sodium soy sauce
- 1 tablespoon Schezuan sauce
- teaspoons cornstarch
- 1 tablespoon canola oil
- 1 lb chicken breast, boneless and cut into 1 inch cubes

Directions:

2. Cook brown rice separately according to package instructions.
3. Take a small bowl and mix together orange juice, sauces, corn starch and set aside for a while.
4. Heat oil in a pan and cook chicken in it until brown. Then add in cabbage, broccoli, peas and sauce mixture from the bowl.
5. Cook on low heat for 20 to 25 minutes until all Ingredients: get tender.
6. Sprinkle sesame seed on top and then serve with brown rice.

Chicken And Wild Rice Stuffed Tomatoes

Ingredients:

- cups uncooked wild rice
- cups vegetable broth, low sodium
- chicken breasts
- large red tomatoes
- 1 tablespoon fresh basil
- cloves garlic, minced
- 1 cup shredded parmesan cheese
- tablespoons olive oil

Directions:

1. First, cook the wild rice according to package instructions using broth instead of water.
2. Meanwhile, preheat oven at 5 75 degree F.
3. Grill the chicken in oven until done and set aside.

4. Center cord the tomatoes by cutting top of it.
5. When rice is cooked, add in the chicken, basil, garlic and cheese
6. Stuff tomatoes with the rice filling and drizzle olive oil on top
7. Keep repeating until all tomatoes are done.
8. Bake in oven for another 15-20 minutes
9. Serve and enjoy.

Fish Tacos

Ingredients:

- 1 onion, chopped
- 1 tablespoon cilantro, chopped
- teaspoons olive oil
- 1/10 teaspoon cayenne pepper optional
- 1/10 teaspoon black pepper
- 1/2 teaspoon salt
- pounds cod fillets
- tablespoons lime juice
- tomatoes, chopped

Coleslaw

- 1 cup nonfat sour cream
- 1 cup of salsa
- 7 of 7 -inch corn tortillas
- 1 cup red cabbage, shredded

- 1 cup green onions, chopped

Directions:

1. Preheat oven to 5 75 degrees.
2. Bake the fish in the oven.
3. Take a bowl and mix lime juice, tomato, cilantro, onion, olive oil, salt and both pepper.
4. Spoon the mixture on fillets
5. In addition, bake again for 12 -20 to 25 minutes
6. Mix red cabbage, onions, sour cream and salsa in bowl.
7. Divide fish among the tortilla and spread a generous amount of slaw mixture on top.
8. Fold and enjoy.

Strawberry And Banana Smoothie

Ingredients:

- 1 and ½ cups non-fat milk
- 1 tablespoon stevia
- 1 banana, peeled and sliced
- strawberries, halved
- ½ teaspoon vanilla extract

Directions:

1. In your blender, mix strawberries with vanilla, milk and banana and pulse well.
2. Divide into glasses and serve right away.

Shrimp And Artichoke Frittata

Ingredients:

- ounces shrimp, peeled, deveined and halved
- eggs
- ounces canned artichokes, drained and chopped
- ¼ cup fat-free milk
- A pinch of black pepper
- A pinch of garlic powder
- ¼ cup green onions, chopped
- Cooking spray
- 1 tablespoons low-fat cheddar, grated
- cherry tomatoes, halved
- tablespoon parsley, chopped

Directions:

1. In a bowl, mix eggs with milk, black pepper, garlic powder and green onions and whisk
2. Grease a pan with the cooking spray, heat it up over medium-high heat, add shrimp, stir and cook for 5 minutes.
3. Add eggs mix, spread, reduce heat to medium, cook until the eggs are done and take off heat.
4. Sprinkle artichokes, cheddar cheese, tomatoes and parsley on top, cover pan, leave aside for 4 minutes, divide frittata between plates and serve for breakfast.

Easy Spinach and Quinoa Pancakes

Ingredients:

- ½ cup low-fat parmesan, grated
- Black pepper to the taste
- ½ teaspoon basil, dried
- 1 cups baby spinach leaves
- 1 cups salsa
- teaspoons olive oil
- 1 and ½ cups water
- garlic cloves, minced
- ¾ cup quinoa
- egg whites

Directions:

1. Put the water in a pan, bring to a boil over medium-high heat, add quinoa and the garlic, stir, cover, simmer for 12 minutes, uncover pan, cook for 3 minutes more, take off heat,

drain, transfer to a bowl, fluff with a fork and cool down.
2. Add parmesan, basil, black pepper and egg whites and whisk everything well.
3. Heat up a pan with half of the oil over medium heat, make 3 pancakes out of the quinoa mix, place them in the pan, cook for 3 minutes on each side and transfer them to a lined baking sheet.
4. Add the rest of the oil to the pan and also heat up over medium-high heat.
5. Make 3 more quinoa pancakes, cook them for 3 minutes on each side and also transfer them to the baking sheet.
6. Introduce pancakes in the oven at 5 50 degrees F for 5 minutes and divide them between plates
7. Serve for breakfast.

Orange Yogurt

Ingredients:

- ounces low-fat yogurt
- 0 ounces strawberries
- 1 cup low-fat milk
- 1 cup orange juice

Directions:

1. In your blender mix orange juice with milk, yogurt and strawberries and whisk well.
2. Divide into 3 glasses and serve.

Easy Shrimp Salad

Ingredients:

For The Shrimp:

- 1 teaspoon Cajun spice
- tablespoons olive oil
- garlic cloves, minced
- 1 pound shrimp, peeled and deveined

For the salad:
- 1 cucumber, sliced
- avocados, peeled, pitted and chopped
- 1 cup corn
- Juice of 1 lemon
- ½ bunch parsley, chopped
- tablespoons olive oil
- cups lettuce leaves, torn
- tomatoes, chopped
- 1 small yellow onion, chopped

- A pinch of black pepper

Direction:

1. In a bowl, combine the shrimp with Cajun spice and garlic and toss.
2. Heat up a pan with 3 tablespoons oil over medium-high heat, add shrimp, cook for 3 minutes on each side and transfer to a bowl.
3. Add lettuce, tomatoes, onion, cucumber, avocado, corn and a pinch of pepper and toss.
4. In a small bowl, mix 3 tablespoons oil with parsley and lemon juice, whisk well, pour over the salad, toss and serve for lunch.

Chicken With Noodles

Ingredients:

- 1 tsp. Basil
- 1 chopped Onion small
- Salt
- Chicken Soup
- cups of Noodles
- Water
- 7 boneless Chicken Legs
- Diced Carrots
- 12 oz Corn frozen
- 12 oz Peas frozen

Directions:

1. In a cooker, place carrots on the bottom.
2. Put the chicken on top of the carrots.
3. Add water and cook on high temp for 12 hrs.
4. Transfer the chicken to a plate.

5   Drain the water.
6   Place the chicken back into the cooker.
7   Now, pour the chicken soup over the chicken along with water 3 cans.
8   Add i basil, corn and onion. Add water to cover the vegetables.
9   Cook for 12 hrs on low.
10 Place noodles in the cooker.
11 Cook again for 3 5 mins on "high".
12 Serve hot.

Chili Con Carne

Ingredients:

For Spice Paste:

- chopped Jalapeño
- 1 tbsp. Water
- 1 tbsp. Cumin
- tsp. Cocoa Powder unsweetened
- 1 Chili Powder
- 1 Chipotle Powder
- tsp. Cornmeal

For Chili:

- 15 ounces Kidney Beans Red
- 15 ounces Northern Beans
- diced Carrots
- cups Chicken Stock
- 1 tbsp. Vegetable Oil

- 15   ounces Beef Sirloin cubed
- 1 chopped Onion large
- cloves Garlic
- 15 ounces Tomatoes diced

Directions:

1. Blend spices and water into a paste in a food processor.
2. Oil a sauté pan.
3. Brown the beef in the pan.
4. Transfer the beef into the slow cooker.
5. Now, place onions the pan.
6. Sauté for at least 5 mins.
7. Pour the spice paste into the pan.
8. Stir well.
9. Transfer the paste mix to the slow cooker.
10. Add the chicken stock.
11. Put remaining Ingredients: in the cooker and cook for 7   hrs. Serve hot.

Chili Beans And Sweet Potato

Ingredients:

- drained Black Beans
- Chili Powder
- tsp. Cocoa Powder
- cloves Garlic
- tsp. Salt
- 1 cup Water
- 1 tbsp. of Cumin
- Olive Oil
- 1 cubed Sweet Potato large
- chopped Carrots small
- oz. Tomatoes, diced with juice

Directions:

1. In a frying pan, cook garlic and onion in oil.

2. Then add salt.
3. Add remaining vegetables.
4. Put the beans in the slow cooker.
5. Put in the onion mixture as well.
6. Cook on "high" for 7 hrs.
7. Stir once and add 1 cup of Water. Cook again for 5 0 mins. Serve hot.

Slow Cooker Chicken Soup

Ingredients:

- Parsley Sprigs
- Thyme Sprigs
- Bay Leaf
- Peppercorns whole
- 1 crushed clove of Garlic
- cups Water
- 1 diced Carrot
- 1 chopped Celery Stalk
- 1 sliced Onion
- pounds Chicken Legs

Directions:

1. Place all the elements in the slow cooker and mix them well
2. Cook on "High" temperature for 4 hrs. Serve hot.

Chicken Cacciatore

Ingredients:

- sliced Onions
- 1 sliced Green Pepper
- oz. Mushroom
- 15 oz. Tomatoes diced
- minced cloves Garlic
- Oregano dried
- Basil dried
- Salt
- Parmesan cheese, shredded
- 1/10 cup of universal Flour
- tbsp. Canola Oil
- broiler Chicken

Directions:

1. Coat chicken with flour by tossing in a plastic bag.
2. Now, brown the chicken in a skillet.
3. Transfer it to the oven.
4. Place the others the ingredient in the oven
5. Heat on "low" temp for 4 hrs.
6. Serve hot after garnishing with Parmesan.

Chicken And Wide Rice Stuffed Tomatoes

Ingredients:

- 1 cup vegetable broth low Sodium
- large tomatoes
- cloves minced garlic
- tablespoon olive oil
- ½ cup parmesan grated cheese
- tablespoon basil
- 1 chicken breast
- 1 cup rice

Directions:

1. Cook rice by following the instruction written on the packet using mixture of water and low sodium vegetable broth.
2. Grill and slice the chicken breast into small pieces.

3. Mix the chicken, garlic, basil and most of the parmesan cheese into the cooked rice; Use the wild rice filling to fill the tomatoes.
4. Garnish it by using the remaining parmesan.
5. At 5 50 degree, brush the tomatoes with the olive oil and cook for 3 0minutes.

Apple-Cinnamon Granola

Ingredients:

- ¼ tsp. ground cardamom
- 1 cup whole-grain toasted oat cereal
- 1 cup chopped apple dried
- 1/10 cup applesauce
- tbsp. butter
- ¼ cup honey
- Cooking spray
- tsp. ground cinnamon
- 1/10 cup oat bran
- cups regular oats
- 1/10 cup finely walnuts chopped

Directions:

1. Preheat oven to 3 50 degree. Mix the first 7 Ingredients: in a bowl and stir.

2. Melt butter in a saucepan over heat. Add honey, brown sugar, 1/10 cup applesauce to pan, and bring to a boil. Cook for a minute, stirring continuously. Mix both the applesauce mixture and oat mixture, stirring to coat. Spread on a jelly-roll pan and bake for at least an hour and 5 0 minutes. Stir in chopped apple after it is cool.
3. Granola should be stored in an airtight container up to one 1 week.

Beef Stroganoff

Ingredients:

- ½ cup sour cream fat-free
- cups uncooked yolkless egg noodles
- ½ lb boneless beef steak
- ½ can fat-free of mushroom soup
- ½ tsp. paprika
- 1 tablespoon plain flour
- ½ cup chopped onion

Directions:

1. Sauté the onions over mind heat until they are translucent.
2. Add the beef and continue cooking for at least 5 minutes. Drain and set aside.
3. Fill a large pot with water ¾ full and allow boiling. Cook the noodles according to the

directions found on the package. Drain the pasta when cooked.

4 Mix the soup and flour together with a little water in a saucepan over mind heat. It should take the sauce about five 5 minutes to thicken.

5 Mix the paprika, beef and soup together and warm thoroughly. Add the sour cream whilst stirring and serve immediately.

Baking Apple

Ingredients:

- teaspoon brown sugar
- ½ cup rum
- teaspoon golden raisins
- Light whipped cream
- Vanilla extract
- fuji
- teaspoon lemon juice

Directions:

1. Heat oven to 550 degree F. Create a core on each apple without cutting through, in order for the bottom to remain intact.
2. Remove at least ½ inch of the peel at the top of each apple.
3. Place them in a baking dish and sprinkle with lemon juice. The centers should be filled with

brown sugar and raisins. Sprinkle with cinnamon and drizzle with vanilla extract.

4   Pour sherry, rum into the bottom of the dish. Bake for 60 minutes. Let stand for 3 minutes, top with light whipped cream.

The Healthy French Toast

Ingredients:

- ½ cup mashed apples
- ½ cup zero fat milk
- 1 spoon of sugar
- slices of whole grain bread
- whole egg
- 1 Pinch of cinnamon

Directions:

1. Mix the milk, egg, cinnamon, mashed apple and cinnamon in a bowl.
2. Soak the bread and make sure the egg-mixture is fully absorbed.
3. Grease the skillet with light butter and cook the bread until it turns golden brown.
4. Serve when food is ready.

Oat Pancakes

Ingredients:

- tablespoon of vegetable oil
- ½ tbsp. maple syrup
- 1 cup of zero fat milk
- 1 spoon of sugar
- ½ cup flour
- ½ cup flour whole wheat
- 1 Pinch of salt
- cup of oat
- 1 eggs

Directions:

1. Blend the oat and mix it with milk, egg, flour, salt and vegetable oil.
2. Coat the skillet with a cooking spray and then heat. Pour ¼ cup of the mixture and cook for 3 to 5   minutes. Cook the other sides following

the same direction and serve with maple syrup and power sugar on top.

Burrito

Ingredients:

- Sea salt
- 1 Pepper
- ½ sliced red pepper
- ¼ cup of diced onion
- 1 teaspoon grape seed oil
- ½ teaspoon cumin
- 1 rice tortilla
- 1 whole egg
- ¼ diced avocado
- 1 tablespoon chopped cilantro

Directions:

1. Heat grape seed oil, onion and pepper in a skillet. Sauté until vegetables are soft. Season with salt, cumin and pepper.

2. Add your eggs and scramble together. Cook for 4 minutes and then add cilantro before the egg is well cooked.
3. Heat up rice tortilla over a low heat. 3 0 seconds on each side until it warmed.
4. Fill the tortilla with diced avocado and the scrambled egg.
5. Then serve.

Ravioli Skillet Lasagna

Ingredients:

- ¼ cup parmesan cheese or grated Romano
- oz. frozen chopped spinach
- cups purchase pasta sauce
- oz. frozen cheese
- 1/10 cup water
- egg
- 30   oz. carton ricotta cheese

Directions:

1. Combine the water and pasta sauce in a 12 inch skillet, put over heat
2. Stir in ravioli. Cook over a medium heat for 5 minutes. Stir once to prevent it from sticking
3. In a medium bowl stir egg, cheese, and ricotta and Romano cheese together. Top ravioli with spinach.

4. Cook over low heat until ricotta layer is set. Sprinkle each serving with additional Romano cheese.

Orange Roast Chicken

Ingredients:

- 1 clove garlic, chopped
- 1 teaspoon rosemary, chopped
- ¼ cup orange juice
- ½ teaspoon olive oil
- Lime juice
- skinless boneless chicken breast

Directions:

1. Coat each chicken with oil and rub garlic into each of the chicken breast. Season with rosemary and pepper
2. Place the in a baking dish, pour over lime juice and orange juice on the chicken
3. Bake for about 5 0 minutes and then turn the chicken and bake for another 12 minutes.

4. The orange juice in the bottom of dish will help prevent it from drying.

Salmon With Broccoli & Red Potatoes

Ingredients:

- 1 tablespoon whole-grain mustard
- 1 tablespoon lemon juice
- 1 tablespoon along with 3 tablespoon olive oil extra virgin
- 1/3 -pound broccoli florets torn into 3 " pieces
- 1/3 -pound small red potatoes unpeeled & halved
- tablespoon honey
- 3 7 oz-12 oz of center-cut without salmon fillets 1 - 1 ½ thick
- tablespoon fresh minced chives
- salt & ground black pepper for taste

Directions:

1 Set the lowest location of the toaster oven rack, pick the convection setting, and heat the oven
2 to 500 °F.
3 . Clean all over with 1 teaspoon oil and spray with 1/2teaspoon salt and 1/2teaspoon pepper. Dry with paper towels. Until required, refrigerate it.
4 . Brush the rimmed baking sheet, with a 1 tablespoon oil toaster oven. Apply 1 tablespoon of oil to the potatoes, season with salt & pepper, and place the cut side down on half of the pan.
5 4. Apply 1   tablespoon of oil to the broccoli, season with salt and pepper and place on the other half of the board. Heat until potatoes are light golden brown and broccoli on the bottom is dark brown for 30 to 35 minutes, rotating the sheet halfway while baking.

6. Meanwhile, mix the chives, mustard, honey, lemon juice, 1 tablespoon of oil left in the bowl, and make a season with the salt and pepper.

7. . Keep it warm, take the sheet from the oven, and pass the bowl's broccoli. To make it browned, cover with foil. Remove any pieces of broccoli left on the sheet by using a spatula. Keep the potatoes on the pan.

8. 7. Place the salmon skin side down on the mat and spread equally. Place the sheet in the oven and reduce the temperature of the oven to 3 75 °F instantly. Bake until the fillet centers reaches at 15 5 °F medium-rare for 25 to 30 minutes, turning the sheet halfway through the baking process. Move the potatoes and salmon to your broccoli platter. Serve with a dressing of chives.

Whole Grain Pasta & Pumpkin Bake

Ingredients:

- 1 cup toasted whole wheat bread-crumbs
- 1 clove garlic peeled
- 1 20 to 25 oz-Can of pumpkin puree unsweetened
- 1 20 to 25 oz-Can of coconut milk
- Kosher salt & cracked black pepper for taste
- 1/4-pound whole-grain penne
- tablespoon paprika

Directions

1. 1. First, heat the oven to 5   50°F.
2. 3 . Put a big pot to boil the water and season with salt liberally. Following the package directions, cook the pasta for 3   minutes. Reserve and set aside 3   cups of pasta water.

Drain the spaghetti, put it in a mixing bowl and set it aside.

3. . In a mixer, mix the coconut milk, ginger, pumpkin puree, salt and plenty of crushed black pepper. Blend until smooth, and add if necessary some pasta water to make it thin. The noodles drain a lot of the sauce, so it should be thin enough to easily pour from the carafe.

4. Pour over the spaghetti with the pumpkin sauce and stir to coat. Cover with breadcrumbs and put in a baking dish. Place for 20 to 25 minutes in the oven until golden brown color appears, bubbling along the edges.

Daphne Oz's Philly Cheesesteak Tacos

Ingredients:

- oregano sprigs/1 teaspoon dried
- 1 teaspoon of Kosher salt
- 1 thinly sliced, cored & seeded red bell pepper
- 1 lb. skirt steak
- 1 halved & thinly sliced medium onion
- 1 cup of low-moisture mozzarella/Monterey jack cheese
- button mushrooms/creminis stemmed by caps-thinly sliced
- 4-7 7 " flour tortillas
- tablespoon butter unsalted
- tablespoon olive oil extra virgin

Directions:

1. Melt butter over medium heat in a medium skillet. Season with salt and pepper on the steak, and transfer to the pan. For medium-rare or longer, sear on both sides for 4 minutes if you want it to cook more. Take the steak out of the pan and let it sit for 12 minutes.
2. Cover the pan with 1 teaspoon of olive oil and add the oregano and onion. To caramelize the onions, simmer for 5 0 minutes over a low flame. Stir in the bell peppers and simmer for about 5 more minutes until they become soft.
3. Take the steak out of the pan and apply the remaining olive oil along with the mushrooms to the pan. Cook until browned and introduce salt to the seasoning.
4. Cut the steak with the mushrooms and add them to the pan. Stir in the peppers and

onions. Top with the cheese and to melt, cover the plate.

5. Heat the tortillas and fill with the top. Now you can serve.

Vegetables And Turkey Stir-Fry

Ingredients:

- 1 tablespoon oil
- 1 cup turkey cut into ½ cubes
- 1 peeled & minced clove garlic/2 tsp garlic powder
- ½ teaspoon sugar
- ½ teaspoon salt
- Thin slices & minced ginger root
- cups cooked brown rice
- cups chopped fresh, canned or frozen vegetables such as mushrooms, bok choy, celery & water chestnuts

Directions:

1. Heat the oil over medium heat in a large skillet. Add the salt, the turkey, the root of ginger, the garlic, and the vegetables. For 1

minute, please do a stir-fry. To avoid scorching, reduce the heat. Only add sugar.

2. Remove the pan from the heat until the vegetables are tender. Add 1-3 tablespoons of water and simmer for 3 more minutes until tender or if the vegetables are still hard. Serve with rice or noodles. Leftovers can be refrigerated within 3 -5 hours.

Pantry Minestrone

Ingredients:

- Kosher salt & cracked black pepper for taste
- cups vegetable /chicken stock low-sodium
- tablespoons of basil pesto
- tablespoons of tomato paste
- tablespoons of olive oil
- cups frozen thawed vegetable medley
- cups frozen thawed broccoli
- cloves sliced garlic
- drained & rinsed-Can of white beans
- 1 sweet potato peeled & diced
- 1 onion diced
- 1 cup Spinach frozen
- 1 bay leaf

- 1 12 oz can of whole peeled tomatoes roughly chopped

Directions:

1. Over medium to high heat, warm up a big Dutch oven or soup pot and add olive oil. Add the onions, garlic, sweet potatoes, and season with salt and pepper when warmed.
2. Add the tomato paste and simmer for an extra 5 minutes. Add the broccoli, Spinach and veggies and cook until it gets warm. Boil and stir in the tomatoes, beans, and stock. Put the bay leaf in and reduce the heat to a low level.
3. For 3 5 to 5 0 minutes, cook. Taste and ladle into bowls for seasoning. Using basil pesto for topping and serve with crusty bread.

Tex-Mex Loaded Baked Sweet Potatoes

Ingredients:

- ½ teaspoon paprika
- 1/10 cups of canned sodium black beans reduced, rinsed and drained
- 1 red pepper diced about ½ cup
- 1 teaspoon of chili powder
- 1 teaspoon of low sodium taco seasoning
- 1 teaspoon of olive oil
- medium-sized potatoes sweet
- Pinch of salt
- ¼ cup cilantro or scallions chopped
- ½ cup Greek yogurt / light sour cream fat-free
- ½ cup Mexican cheese blend reduced fat
- ½ cup salsa non-compulsory

- ½ red onion diced about ½ cup
- ½ teaspoon cumin

Directions:

1. Poke holes with a fork in the potato, cook on the potato setting of your microwave until the potatoes are soft and cooked through for 4 potatoes, around 12 -12 minutes on high. Cook in the oven for around 45 minutes at 400 °F, if you don't have a microwave.
2. In a shallow bowl, add the yogurt and taco seasoning and meld well.
3. Heat oil over low heat in a medium pot. Add the peppers, chili powder, onions, paprika, salt and cumin and simmer for around 5 minutes until the onions are gently caramelized.
4. Now include black beans and mix to blend and heat approximately for 5 more minutes.
5. Cut down the potato lengthwise or use a fork to pierce the surface.

6. Cover with 1/10 cup of black bean blend, 3 tablespoons of shredded cheese, 3 tablespoons of Greek yogurt blend and 3 tablespoons of salsa.

Tandoori Chicken

Ingredients:

- 1 teaspoon yellow curry powder
- 1 teaspoon ground ginger
- 1 teaspoon red pepper flakes - crushed use ½ teaspoon for a milder flavor
- 1 cup plain yogurt nonfat
- ½ cup lemonade
- boneless, skinless chicken breasts
- skewers 5 crushed garlic cloves
- tablespoon paprika

Directions:

1. 1st heat the oven to 400 °F. In a blender, combine the milk, garlic, lemon juice, ginger, yellow curry powder, red pepper flakes and paprika and mix smoothly.

2. Onto each of the soaked skewers, skewer the equivalent number of chicken bits. Place the chicken skewers in a shallow casserole dish. Add half of a mixture of yogurt, and reserved the rest. Cover for about 20 to 25 minutes and cool.

3. With cooking sauce, spray another small baking dish. Remove the chicken skewers, dispose of the marinade with the yogurt, and put the chicken skewers in the bowl. Brush the chicken with a blend of reserved yogurt.

4. Bake for 20 to 30 minutes or until juices run clear when meat is pierced. Instantly serve. Grill the chicken, skewers over medium-high heat for 6-10 minutes on either hand for much more authentic preparation.

Turkey Fajitas Bowls

Ingredients:

- 1 lb. turkey breast
- large piece yellow bell pepper cut into 1' piece
- 1 big green pepper cut into 1' piece
- 1 cup cheddar cheese shredded for topping
- 1 tbsp lemon juice
- 1 medium tomato pierce into 15 wedges
- 1 crushed clove Garlic
- tablespoons salsa for topping
- 4- 12 inches corn tortillas or you can make your particular tostada bowls
- /4 tsp fresh chile pepper or dried for taste
- tsp olive oil
- 1 tsp dried oregano leaves

Directions:

1. Tear the turkey into thin slices and then into 5 /4-inch short strips. Add 1 tablespoon of oil with garlic, lemon juice, oregano and chili pepper in a medium dish. Add the turkey and stir for coating. Let it marinate for half an hour.
2. Heat the remaining 1 tbsp oil in a nonstick skillet at medium-high heat. Stir in the yellow and green peppers and fry for 3 minutes. Add the turkey strips and fry for an extra 5 minutes. Heat the tomatoes and stir.
3. In a pan, hot tortillas are used as a basis. Pour in the bowl of tortilla or tostada and top with salsa and cheese.

Sesame-Honey Chicken & Quinoa Bowl

Ingredients:

Quinoa And Carrot Slaw:

- 1 tbsp rice vinegar
- tbsp toasted sesame seeds
- 1 tbsp sesame oil
- /4 cup quinoa, rinsed
- 1 & 1   cup water
- 1 cups of grated carrots approximately 5 large

Sesame-Honey Chicken:

- tablespoons water
- tbsp sesame oil
- scallions sliced
- cups prepared chicken breast pierce into the bite-sized pieces

- 1 teaspoon cornstarch
- tablespoons reduced-sodium soy sauce
- tablespoons honey

Directions:

1. To make the quinoa: Boil 1½ cups of water in a shallow saucepan. Add the quinoa and put it to a boil again. Reduce to a medium boil, cover and cook for 12 to 15 minutes before the water is absorbed. Uncover them and wait.
2. Meanwhile, in a medium dish, mix the rice vinegar, carrots, rice vinegar, seeds, sesame and 1 tablespoon of the oil. Put it aside.
3. Combine the soy sauce, sesame oil, sugar, and cornstarch 3 teaspoons of water in a shallow cup. Pour it into a medium skillet. Cook and stir over medium heat until the sauce becomes thickened. Add the chicken and stir for about 1 minute before it is coated with the sauce.

4. Divide the quinoa and top each with 1 cup of carrot slaw and 5 /4 cup of chicken mixture in 4 cups. Sprinkle with green onion.

Southwest Tortilla Bake

Ingredients:

- 1 tsp chili powder
- 1 tomato sliced
- 1 cup Monterey Jack cheese shredded
- 1 cup fresh / frozen corn
- 1 cup milk fat-free
- 1 cup of cooked black / pinto beans
- 1 4-ounce can green chilies diced
- 1 Salsa
- Eight corn tortillas cut in half
- eggs
- green onions sliced

Directions:

1. 1st heat the oven up to 5 50 °F.

2. Using nonstick spray or oil to coat an 12 - inch square baking dish. Arrange 5 tortilla halves to line the bottom of the plate. Top each of cheese, corn and beans with 1/10 of a cup. Utilize 1 of the green onions to sprinkle. To layer and top with beans, 1/10 cup cheese, the leftover corn, and green onions, place a further 5 tortilla halves on top. To shield, place the last 5 tortilla pieces over the corner.
3. Add the eggs, chili powder and milk to a medium bowl and whisk to mix. Stir in the chilies. Pour the egg and milk mixture equally over the tortillas. Top with both the 1/10 cup of left cheese and tomato slices.
4. Uncovered and bake for about 50 minutes until a knife inserted in the middle. Let it stand at room temperature for 12 minutes before serving. Serve hot with salsa.

Flank Steak And Roasted Corn Salad With Vinaigrette

Ingredients:

- Fresh cilantro chopped ¼ cup
- Ground cumin 1 tablespoon
- Dried oregano 3 teaspoons
- Red pepper flakes ¼ teaspoon
- Flank steak ¾ pound
- Romaine lettuce 1 large head
- Cherry tomatoes halved 4 cups
- Red onion thinly sliced ¾ cup
- Black beans cooked 1 ½ cups
- Fresh corn kernels 5 cups
- Water ½ cup
- Fresh lime juice 3 tablespoons
- Red bell pepper chopped 3 tablespoons

- Olive oil extra-virgin 3 tablespoons
- Salt ½ teaspoon
- Black pepper freshly ground ½ teaspoon

Directions:

1. Begin by trimming the romaine lettuce and tearing it into bite-sized pieces.
2. Place a large cast-iron pan on a medium-high flame and add in the corn. Dry roast for about 5 minutes. Continue stirring to prevent the kernels from burning. Once done, set aside.
3. Take a blender and add in the water, bell pepper, lime juice, and a cup of roasted corn. Blend into a smooth puree-like consistency.
4. Now add the olive oil, cilantro, ¼ teaspoon of salt, and ¼ teaspoon of black pepper to the blender. Blend

again until you have a smooth puree-like consistency. Set aside.
5. Prepare a charcoal grill by starting a fire. Take the grill rack and lightly coat it with the cooking spray. Place the grill rack 7 inches from the fire.
6. Take a small mixing bowl and add in the cumin, red pepper flakes, oregano, remaining salt, and remaining black pepper. Mix well.
7. Place the steak in a shallow dish and sprinkle the prepared spice mix. Rub it evenly on both sides.
8. Place the steak on the grill rack and cook for 5 minutes; flip over and cook for another 5 minutes. Once done, set aside to cool for at least 5 minutes.
9. Slice the steak into ¼-inch slices and set aside.

10. Take a large mixing bowl and add in the lettuce, onion, tomatoes, 5 cups of roasted corn, and black beans. Toss well to combine the ingredients.
11. Pour the prepared vinaigrette over the veggies and mix gently until all Ingredients: are evenly coated.
12. Serve the prepared salad on the plates and serve each plate with sliced steak.

Chicken Salad Grilled With Buttermilk Dressing

Ingredients:

For Dressing:

- Fresh dill finely chopped 3 tablespoons
- Garlic minced 1 teaspoon
- Black pepper cracked as per taste
- Mayonnaise fat-free 1/10 cup
- Buttermilk low-fat ¼ cup

For Salad:

- Salad greens torn 12 cups
- Red bell pepper sliced 1
- Sweet onion sliced ½
- Chicken breasts boneless and skinless 4
- Olive oil extra-virgin 3 teaspoons

Directions:

1. Begin by taking a small bowl and adding in the buttermilk, mayonnaise, garlic, black pepper, and dill. Use a whisk to mix the Ingredients: well and transfer into a glass bowl. Cover it with a lid. Place the dressing in the refrigerator.
2. Prepare the charcoal grill and light the fire. Take the grill rack and lightly grease it with cooking spray. Place the greased rack 7 inches over the fire.
3. Place the chicken breasts on a shallow dish and brush them generously with olive oil. Place the chicken breasts onto the grill.
4. Grill the chicken breasts for 5 minutes; flip over and cook for another 5 minutes.
5. Once done, transfer the grilled chicken breasts to a chopping block for 5 minutes. Once the chicken is done resting, cut it into thin slices.

6. Take a large mixing bowl and add in the salad greens, onion, and bell pepper. Drizzle ¾ of the buttermilk dressing. Toss until all veggies are evenly coated.
7. Transfer about 3 cups of salad on each of the plates and place the sliced chicken on top.
8. Finish with a final drizzle of buttermilk dressing.
9. Serve right away!

Chicken Burritos

Ingredients:

- Fresh oregano 3 tablespoons
- Garlic chopped 3 cloves
- Chicken breasts cooked 12 ounces
- Tortillas whole-wheat 4 12-inch diameter
- Canned black beans drained and rinsed ½ cup
- Green cabbage shredded 3 cups
- Oil 1 teaspoon
- Red bell pepper finely chopped 1
- Jalapeno pepper seeded and finely chopped 1
- Celery ribs chopped 3
- Yellow onion finely chopped 1
- Cumin seed 3 tablespoons
- Grape tomatoes 3 cups

Directions:

- Take a large nonstick skillet and place it on a medium-high flame.
- Pour in the oil and let it heat through. Toss in the onion, celery, cumin, and pepper. Sauté for around 20 to 25 minutes. Continue stirring to prevent the Ingredients: from sticking to the bottom.
- Now add in the tomatoes, garlic, and oregano and continue to cook for another 12 minutes.
- Transfer the Ingredients: to a blender and blend into a smooth puree-like consistency.
- Place the cooked chicken breasts onto a plate and use a fork to pull the chicken apart.
- Place the tortillas on a flat surface and begin assembling. Top each tortilla with an equal amount of pulled chicken. Top the chicken with cabbage, beans, and the sauce.

- Roll the tortillas into burritos. Enjoy and serve right away!

Brussels Sprouts With Lemon And Shallots

Ingredients:

- Brussels sprouts 1 pound
- Vegetable stock no salt added ½ cup
- Lemon zest finely grated ¼ teaspoon
- Fresh lemon juice 1 tablespoon
- Black pepper freshly ground ¼ teaspoon
- Olive oil extra-virgin 5 teaspoons
- Shallots thinly sliced 5 small
- Salt divided ¼ teaspoon

Directions:

1. Start by trimming the Brussels sprouts and cutting them into quarters.
2. Take a large cast-iron pan and place it on a medium-high flame. Pour in a couple of teaspoons of olive oil.

3. Add in the finely sliced shallots and keep stirring to sauté for around 7 minutes. Make sure the shallots are golden and not caramelized. Sprinkle ⅛ teaspoon of salt over the shallots and stir. Once done, transfer the shallots into a small bowl and set aside.
4. Return the pan to the flame and add in the remaining teaspoon of olive oil.
5. Toss in the quartered Brussels sprouts and cook for about 4 minutes. Keep stirring to prevent them from caramelizing.
6. Pour in the vegetable stock and let it simmer. Cook for about 7 minutes or until the Brussels sprouts are tender.
7. Return the sautéed shallots to the Brussels sprouts and vegetable stock. Add in the lemon juice and lemon zest. Stir well.
8. Finish by seasoning the Brussels sprouts with ⅛ teaspoon of freshly ground pepper. Mix well. Serve and enjoy!

Barley And Tomato Roast Risotto

Ingredients:

- Shallots chopped 3
- Dry white wine ¼ cup
- Pearl barley 3 cups
- Fresh basil chopped 5 tablespoons
- Fresh flat-leaf parsley chopped 5 tablespoons
- Fresh thyme chopped 1 ½ tablespoons
- Parmesan cheese grated ½ cup
- Plum tomatoes 12 large
- Olive oil extra-virgin 3 tablespoons
- Salt ½ teaspoon
- Black pepper freshly ground ½ teaspoon
- Vegetable stock low-sodium 4 cups
- Water 5 cups

Directions:

1. Begin by preheating the oven by setting the temperature to 450 degrees Fahrenheit.
2. Take a large pan full of water and let it boil. Now add in the tomatoes and boil for about 5 minutes.
3. Take another bowl and fill it with cold water. Once the tomatoes are done, drop the tomatoes into the cold water.
4. Use a knife to peel the skin off the tomatoes and cut them into quarters. Set aside.
5. Take a nonstick baking dish and arrange the tomatoes in a single layer. Drizzle them with a tablespoon of olive oil and season them with ¼ teaspoon salt and pepper. Toss the tomatoes gently.
6. Place the baking sheet in the oven and roast for about 5 0 minutes. Once done, remove

the baking sheet and keep 17 of the tomato wedges for garnishing.

7. Take a large cast-iron pan and place it on a high flame. Add in the water and vegetable stock and let it come to a boil. Reduce the flame to low and let it simmer.

8. Take another heavy saucepan and place it on a medium flame. Pour 1 tablespoon of olive oil and let it heat through.

9. Toss in the shallots and cook for about 5 minutes. Keep stirring to prevent the shallots from caramelizing.

10. Pour in the white wine to deglaze the pan and cook for about 5 minutes or until the liquid is almost evaporated.

11. Now add in the barley and stir well. Cook for about a minute. Stir in about ½ cup of vegetable stock and water mixture. Mix well and let it cook. Once the liquid is absorbed, add ½ cup more of the stock mixture and

repeat the same until the mixture is finished. This will take about 50 minutes.

12. Once the barley is done cooking, turn off the flame and add in the chopped basil, roasted tomatoes, grated cheese, thyme, and parsley. Fold them gently.
13. Season the barley with the remaining pepper and salt. Mix until all Ingredients: are well combined.
14. Transfer the risotto into a serving bowl and garnish with basil leaves and reserved roasted tomatoes.
15. Serve right away!

Chia Pudding

Ingredients:

- cups almond milk
- ½ cup chia seeds
- ¼ cup coconut, shredded
- ¼ cup almonds
- teaspoons coconut sugar

Directions:

1. Put chia seeds in your instant pot, add coconut, almonds, sugar and milk, stir, cover, cook on High for 5 minutes, divide into bowls and serve.

Chicken Vegetable Bake

Ingredients:

- 2 cup all-purpose flour
- 3 tsp *salt*
- 3 tsp dried thyme (crushed)
- 2 tsp black pepper
- 35 cups low–fat or fat–free milk
- 3 cup chopped spinach
- 35 cups cooked white or brown rice
- 3 cups chopped chicken
- 3 cup shredded Parmesan cheese
- 3 cups sliced mushrooms (washed and de-stemmed)
- 3 cup yellow and red bell pepper (Alternatively you can choose sweet peppers)
- 3 onion (finely chopped)

- 3 cloves garlic (peel, wash and mince)
- 3 tbsp olive oil

Directions:

1. Preheat the oven to 310 degrees Fahrenheit.
2. Place a skillet on medium heat and add olive oil to it, add onions and garlic to
3. the skillet. Cook the Ingredients: until the onions have turned golden brown
4. and soft.
5. Now, add the mushroom slices and mixed peppers to the skillet and cook until
6. the mushrooms have released their juices. Continue to cook until the
7. mushroom slices are soft.
8. Add the thyme, flour, salt and black pepper. Stir the Ingredients: well until the
9. mixture is well balanced. Adjust the seasoning if necessary.
10. Pour the milk slowly into the skillet while continuously stirring. Bring the

11. Ingredients: in the skillet to a boil.
12. Now, add the chicken, spinach and rice to the skillet and stir well. Stir the
13. Ingredients: until the chopped chicken is coated well with the sauce.
14. Add the cheese to the skillet and continue to cook until the cheese has melted.
15. Coat the insides of a baking dish with cooking spray and transfer the mixture
16. in the skillet into the dish.
17. Cover the dish and bake for fifteen minutes while it is covered. Then uncover
18. the dish and bake for five more minutes or until the dish is fully cooked.
19. Serve hot.

Onion Omelette

Ingredients:

- 3 cup red onion
- 3 eggs
- 1/2 tsp salt
- 1/2 tsp black pepper
- 3 tablespoon olive oil
- 1/2 cup cheese
- 1/2 tsp basil

Directions:

2. In a bowl combine all Ingredients: together and mix well
3. In a skillet heat olive oil and pour the egg mixture
4. Cook for 3 to 4 minutes per side
5. When ready remove omelette from the skillet and serve

Olive Omelette

Ingredients:

- 2 cup olives
- 2 eggs
- 1/2 tsp salt
- 1/2 tsp black pepper
- 3 tablespoon olive oil
- 1/2 cup cheese
- 1/2 tsp basil

Directions:

1. In a bowl combine all Ingredients: together and mix well
2. In a skillet heat olive oil and pour the egg mixture
3. Cook for 3 to 4 minutes per side
4. When ready remove omelette from the skillet and serve

Tomato Omelette

Ingredients:

- 3 tablespoon olive oil
- 1/2 cup cheese
- 1/2 tsp basil
- 3 cup tomatoes
- 3 eggs
- 1/2 tsp salt
- 1/2 tsp black pepper

Directions:

1. In a bowl combine all Ingredients: together and mix well
2. In a skillet heat olive oil and pour the egg mixture
3. Cook for 3 to 5 minutes per side
4. When ready remove omelette from the skillet and serve